#TTC

Trying to Conceive

YummyYoniPearls.net
Written by Jared & Mesi James

Introduction

The purpose of this guide is to offer tips and information for women who are struggling to conceive naturally or suffer from miscarriages. With the help of Yummy Yoni Pearls, Black Seed Oil, Steam N' Baths, and a better diet, many women have been able to conceive. Yummy Yoni Pearls have been a source of conceiving and birthing over 100 healthy babies within a few years. While cleansing with Yummy Yoni Pearls, plus the one-on-one guidance offered, several women who have been TTC for months or years have been successful.

Although each woman is different, most women suffer from tubular blockage, cyst, fibroids, or irregular cycles, which may cause infertility. However, issues such as chronic BV or abnormal cervical cells can also cause infertility. This guide will provide general information about the reproductive organs, contraception, common causes of infertility, menstruation, ovulation, and tips to conceive with natural herbs. All the products suggested are 100% natural, organic, effective and available online at YummyYoniPearls.net.

Table of Contents

Introduction .... *ii*

Female Reproductive System *1*

Menstruation & Ovulation *5*

Menstruation *6*

Ovulation *8*

More Common Causes Of Irregular Or Absent Periods... *11*

Herbalism *15*

What are Yummy Yoni Pearls? *17*

Success stories with Yummy Yoni Pearls ... *21*

Black Seed Oil #Lifeinacan........................ *23*

Tips To Conceive Naturally *25*

Yummy Yoni Mommies & Babies!............... *29*

Female Reproductive System

Yes, everybody knows that eggs and sperm are needed to make a baby. However, we need to examine the basics in greater detail! First, we will start by taking a guided tour of the reproductive systems of women. The sexual and reproductive organs on the outside of the body are called the external genitals. Around the genital area, there are three openings. In front is the urethra, from where urine comes out; below this is the opening to the vagina, which is called the introitus; and the third is the anus, from where a bowel movement leaves the body.

The outer genital area is called the vulva. The vulva includes the clitoris, the labia majora, and the labia minora. The most sensitive part of the genital area is the clitoris. This is a pea-sized organ that's full of nerve endings since its only purpose is to provide sexual pleasure. The clitoris is protected by a hood of skin and is the equivalent of the man's penis. Feel free to sit down in front of a mirror to get better acquainted with your vagina!

The labia majora, or outer lips, surround the opening to the vagina. They are made of fatty tissue that cushions and protects the vaginal opening. Between these outer lips are labia minora or inner lips. These are sensitive to sexual pleasure. As they are stimulated, they get deeper in color and swell. The vagina is a muscular tunnel that connects the uterus to the outside of the body. It provides an exit for the menstrual fluid and an entrance for the semen.

Normally flat, like a collapsed balloon, the vagina can stretch to accommodate a tampon, a penis, or a baby's head. The walls of the vagina are muscular, smooth and soft. The vagina is a closed space which ends at your cervix. The uterus, or the womb, is the place where the fertilized egg grows and develops during pregnancy. The uterus lies deep in the lower abdomen—the pelvis—and is just behind the urinary bladder. It is a hollow organ shaped like a pear and is about the size of the fist.

Inside the muscular walls of the uterus is a very rich lining—the endometrium—and it is in this lining that the fertilized egg implants. If pregnancy does not occur, the lining is shed along with blood as the menstrual flow. The neck of the uterus is called the cervix, which connects the uterus to the vagina and contains special glands called crypts that make mucus which helps to keep bacteria out of the uterus. The cervical mucus also helps sperms to enter the uterus when the egg is ripe.

The two fallopian tubes are attached to the upper part of the uterus on either side and are about 10 cm long. They are about as big as a piece of spaghetti. Each tube forms a narrow passageway that opens like a funnel into the abdominal cavity, near the ovaries. The ends of the fallopian tubes are draped over the two ovaries, and they serve as a passageway for the egg to travel from the ovary into the uterus. The tube is lined with millions of tiny hairs called cilia that beat rhythmically to propel the egg forward. Of course, the tube is not just a pathway; it performs other functions too, including nourishing the egg and the early embryo in its cavity. Also, the sperm fertilizes the egg in one of the fallopian tubes.

Female Reproductive System

The two almond-sized ovaries are perched in the pelvis, one on each side, just within the fallopian tubes' grasp. The ovary serves two functions: the production of eggs and the secretion of hormones. Each month, at the time of ovulation, a mature egg is released by an ovary. This is 'picked up' by the fimbria and drawn into the fallopian tubes. The eggs in the ovary are stored in follicles (or folliculitis, meaning sack in Latin). These cellular sacks contain the eggs as well as granulosa cells and theca cells which nurture the egg and produce the female hormones.

The ovary has about 2 million eggs during fetal life. From that point onwards, the number of eggs progressively decreases until only about 300,000 eggs are left at the time of birth—a lifetime's stock. During the fertile years, fewer than 500 of these eggs will be released into the fallopian tubes—once in each menstrual cycle. Unlike the testis which is continually churning out billions of new sperm, the ovary never produces any new eggs. One of the existing eggs is matured for ovulation each month, and this limited supply starts what is described as menopause.

The reproductive dance of a female is much different from that of a male. However, the womb is the source of life! A baby develops within the loving care of the womb. For 9 months, a female's body will nurture this new life from the beginning to birth! The vagina has an amazing ability to carry and give life. Unfortunately, some women continue to struggle with irregular cycles and miscarriages. Next, we will examine the importance of the menstrual cycle and ovulation, which are two major causes of infertility in most women trying to conceive.

Menstruation & Ovulation

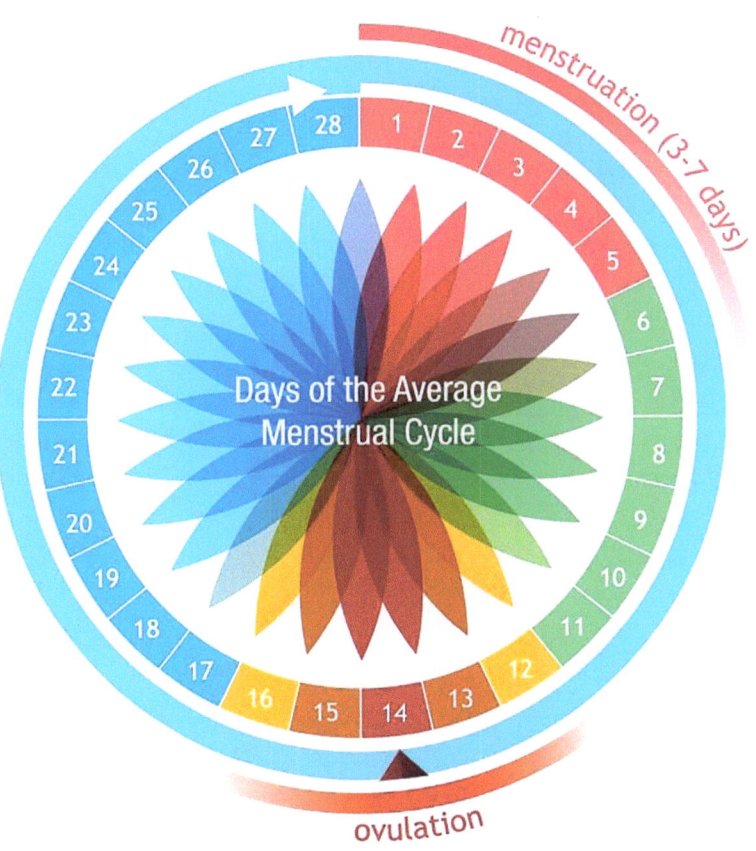

Menstruation

Most women are led to believe that a common menstrual cycle is 3-7 days. However, during research, we discovered that a normal cycle should only be a few minutes to 4 days at the most. Many women suffer from long or heavy cycles for several reasons. Birth control (IUD, Depo Shot, The Pill) can also affect our bodies negatively. While the goal may be not to conceive, some women use birth control to start, stop, or lighten their cycles as well.

The aspect of the reproductive system that women are most aware of is the monthly menstrual cycle. While some women enjoy the idea of not having a period, it is critical for vaginal health. The menstrual cycle is the time from the beginning of one period to the beginning of the next one. Usually, menstrual cycles last about 28–35 days, though anywhere from 3 to 6 weeks is considered common in most females. However, during the menstrual cycle, the uterus is preparing for pregnancy.

Under the influence of the hormones estrogen and progesterone, its lining grows rich and thick to prepare for the fertilized egg. If pregnancy doesn't occur, the uterus must get rid of this lining so that it can grow a new one for the next cycle. The old lining passes out of the uterus through the vagina as the menstrual flow. The menstrual flow may consist of:

- Uterine lining
- Blood clots, which are large portions of the uterine lining as it is released

Menstruation & Ovulation

- Blood released from the blood vessels, which are torn when the uterine lining is released
- Degenerated unfertilized egg

However, as stated previously, some women do not have a period for reasons known and unknown. For example, women who are diagnosed with PCOS, which is Polycystic Ovarian Syndrome, may not see their periods for months or years. The U.S. Department of Health and Human Services estimates around one in twenty women in their childbearing years, in addition to one in ten women (11-years of age and older), are struggling with PCOS. According to these estimates, there are a total of 5 million women in America affected by Polycystic Ovarian Syndrome.

Ovulation

The most effective time to have sex in order to conceive is during the fertile window. The fertile window can last up to six days every month. These six days are the five days leading up to, and the day of, ovulation. Once a month, an egg will mature within one of the two ovaries. As the egg matures, it is released by the ovary, entering the fallopian tube. The egg approaches the sperm waiting and the uterus. The point of ovulation is to have the sperm waiting to fertilize the maturing egg to create a new life. The timing is key.

An egg can survive for roughly 12 hours to a day once released. However, sperm can survive for 5-7 days inside the vagina. Therefore, a six-day window is present for sperm to wait for an egg. Ovulation is affected by several factors, including stress. If you're trying to conceive, we suggest avoiding stressful situations, especially the pressures to conceive. The stressors of trying to conceive can affect women physically and emotionally.

Still, a woman or the 'wombman' is designed perfectly to prepare and give birth. The chances of conceiving are higher during ovulation, especially if you have sex within a day or so of ovulation. When trying to conceive, we suggest downloading a period tracker app, available on most electronic devices. Period tracker apps are a great free tool to help women trying to conceive. A well designed period tracker app can accurately keep track of your fertile window during each cycle. Users can sometimes add additional information such as their body temperature to better predict ovulation.

Women also utilize ovulation test strips, which can detect a spike in luteinizing hormone or (LH). The increase is this particular hormone occurs 24–48 hours before ovulation. A small trace of LH in your blood and urine is normal. However, one or two days before ovulation, it will increase five times the normal amount. The moment your fertile window is open, take advantage of trying to conceive.

Regardless of how long or short your cycle normally is, ovulation usually occurs about 14 days before your next period starts. If you have a 28-day menstrual cycle, you're likely to ovulate around the middle of your cycle. If you have a short cycle, you could ovulate within days of your period ending. If your menstrual cycle is different from one month to the next, your fertile window may also vary by about a week between each period. The core concept of trying to conceive is scheduling intercourse during the ovulation period.

Unfortunately, women cannot conceive without ovulating. Not all women ovulate every month. If an ovary does not produce a mature follicle, ovulation cannot occur. The endometrium or the lining of your uterus will thicken in preparation for pregnancy—as we previously discussed—but no egg is released. Therefore, having a period does not automatically mean that ovulation occurred. Some women may experience an anovulatory cycle, which means ovulation has not occurred. During an anovulatory cycle, women may experience some bleeding, which can appear to be a period, although this is actually not.

Other less common causes of fertility problems in women include blocked fallopian tubes due to pelvic inflammatory disease, endometriosis, or surgery for an ectopic pregnancy, and abnormal uterus. Also, uterine fibroids, which are non-cancerous clumps of tissue and muscle on the walls of the uterus, can cause infertility. Male, not female, infertility is also a growing issue. For instance, a low sperm count can be an issue with conceiving.

However, many men can reverse to a healthy lifestyle. Men reduce the health or number of sperm with heavy alcohol use, drugs, cigarettes, age, or other health problems like cystic fibrosis, which often causes infertility in men. Other related health problems due to hormonal issues or certain cancers can also affect male fertility. Also, for example, cystic fibrosis often causes infertility in men. Infertility in men is most often caused by varicocele, which is when the veins on a man's testicle(s) are too large. Also, exposure to extreme heat can affect the number or shape of the sperm.

More Common Causes Of Irregular Or Absent Periods

Menstrual disorders can cause absent, irregular cycles or spotting. Also, missing menstrual cycles or changes can signal underlying vaginal conditions, which could turn into long-term health consequences. The brain (specifically the hypothalamus and pituitary gland), ovaries, and uterus help to prepare the body for pregnancy. Follicle-stimulating hormone (FSH) and luteinizing hormone (LH) are made by the pituitary gland. Two other hormones, progesterone and estrogen, are made by the ovaries. Menstrual cycle disorders can result from conditions that affect the hypothalamus, pituitary gland, ovaries, uterus, cervix, or vagina.

The section of #TTC will explore the main causes of absent or infrequent cycles. Most causes discussed are based on hormones. Hormonal imbalances or the overproduction of certain hormones can lead to vaginal issues other than absent or irregular cycles. Let's examine more causes of irregular or absent cycles such as Ovarian Failure and the most common causes of infertility—PCOS.

Normally, Ovarian Failure occurs around the age of 50, commonly called menopause. If ovulation stops before age 40, this disorder is called premature ovarian failure or primary ovarian insufficiency. As discussed previously in #TTC, a decrease in hormones can cause absent periods, resulting in infertility. Again, hormonal imbalance is the main cause of early menopause and premature ovarian failure. Now we will discuss the most common reason for infertility—PCOS.

What is Polycystic Ovarian Syndrome (PCOS) exactly? PCOS is described as an uncommon hormonal imbalance. Basically, women with PCOS have an overproduction of androgens or male hormones. This hormonal imbalance or surplus of androgen can cause excessive hair growth, negative skin reactions, and irregular periods. High levels of androgen lead to issues with ovulating and releasing a fertilized egg. Women with PCOS are juggling a variety of issues, including growing cysts in or on the ovaries, which diminishes the chances of conceiving.

Moreover, ovarian cysts, which are said to be normal, can also cause infertility. Some women with or without PCOS can develop fluid-filled sacs in the ovary, commonly formed during ovulation each month. Ovarian cysts can result in abnormal ovulation, and according to the American Society for Reproductive Medicine, ovulation dysfunction accounts for 25 percent of female infertility cases. However, most women with ovarian cysts don't have symptoms. The cysts are usually harmless, which are referred to as functional cysts.

Functional cysts, such as follicular cysts, are the most common type of ovarian cyst. Functional cysts form during a normal menstrual cycle and don't cause or contribute to infertility. However, cysts can become infected and cause a pelvic infection, which could lead to scarring in the fallopian tubes, causing infertility as well. However, this occurrence is extremely rare. Unless the cyst becomes large, these types of ovarian cysts don't affect fertility.

More Common Causes Of Irregular Or Absent Periods

Functional cysts usually go away on their own. However, some cysts don't, which again are caused by hormonal imbalances. For instance, a follicular cyst develops each month and contains the egg inside. The sac ruptures during ovulation, and the egg leaves the ovary. Most follicular cysts will disappear in 2–8 weeks and do not cause pain. However, large cysts may take longer to resolve. Ovarian cysts can result in abnormal ovulation, and according to the American Society for Reproductive Medicine, ovulation dysfunction accounts for 25 percent of female infertility cases.

A normal ovary is about the size of an almond, but if the egg is not ejected, the amount of fluid continues to increase. These types of cyst can reach sizes of up to 10 cm. Fortunately, most follicular cysts are smaller and will resolve within one to three months. Vaginal issues like PCOS also reflect negativity on another important factor to conceive like ovulation. Ovulation during any given cycle depends on the length and regularity of the menstrual cycle. The menstrual cycle of each woman varies.

Some women who suffer from PCOS or endometriosis may suffer from irregular, absent, or painful cycles. Endometriosis is another vaginal issue that can also cause infertility and extreme pain. Endometriosis is usually very painful because the tissue that normally lines the inside of your uterus, or the endometrium, is growing outside of the uterus. Endometriosis commonly affects the ovaries, fallopian tubes, and the tissue lining the pelvis.

Moreover, the excessive endometrial tissue continues to breaks down and bleed with each menstrual cycle. Since the vagina is unable to flush this tissue, the build-up becomes trapped inside the vagina, which can cause abdominal pain. The first symptom many women experience with endometriosis is extremely painful periods. The pain of periods for a woman with 'endo' can reach the point of hospitalization. Women with endometriosis can eventually develop endometrioma, which is when endometrial tissue attaches to the ovary and forms a growth. Also, the severe pelvic pains associated with endo can worsen during menstruation.

However, aren't women told that heavy, painful cycles are normal? Isn't it true that most women suffer from awful periods? The menstrual cycle is notorious for being 7 days of painful bleeding and cramps. However, as mentioned earlier in this guide, periods aren't supposed to be heavy, painful, or long. Some women experience pains before and even after the bleeding has stopped. According to recent information released, endometriosis and PCOS are the two most common vaginal diseases missed by doctors.

The role of the menstrual cycle is imperative in trying to conceive. However, when the information surrounding the 'myths' of the 'red monster' has been altered, abnormalities become the norm. Therefore, what many women do not know as a 'vaginal disorder' or 'hormonal imbalance' is perceived as infertility. A woman's fertility is a precious gift. Unfortunately, many are unable to start the conception process without a regular period.

Herbalism

A regular period helps to balance the harmony of the functioning vagina. The importance of the menstrual cycle goes hand in hand with ovulation. Both are the two main causes of infertility. As stated before, many women experience hormonal imbalances which can affect the menstruation cycle and ovulation. To reverse these issues, simple solutions do exist. Without surgeries or chemicals, women can balance their hormones naturally—with herbalism.

Also known as phytotherapy, herbalism is the study of botany or herbs. Simply put, herbalism is the use of plants for medicinal purposes. Much of modern western medicine originally used plants before being cut with chemicals. Now, prescription drugs, which first derived from plants with medicinal properties, have transformed the pharmaceutical industry. Little to no herbs plants are used to treat medical conditions nowadays.

The typical 'modern' medicine aims to treat one issue. Herbalism, on the other hand, treats the person as a whole with plants that offer therapeutic properties. Herbalism has existed for centuries literally. Some evidence of herbalism dates back more than 60,000 years or 600 CENTURIES. Although herbalism is referred to as an 'alternative therapy,' herbalism in one way, shape, or form is the most common type of medicine practiced worldwide. More than 80 percent of the global population depends on the use of herbs for their health.

YummyYoniPearls.net | Written by Jared & Mesi James

Yummy Yoni Pearls are a form of herbalism, using a particular blend of dried herbs to create a recipe to increase womb health. We will discuss how Yummy Yoni Pearls and other James & James, LLC, products have helped women conceive after months or years of #TTC.

What are Yummy Yoni Pearls?

Yummy Yoni Pearls are cloth-covered balls containing herbs like motherwort, osthol, angelica, borneol, and rhizome. The combination of herbs detoxes your womb and resets your natural balance, increasing elasticity, regulating the menstrual cycle, killing parasites and bacteria, improving fertility, reducing discharge, and removing toxins.

The western medical professional has led women to believe that doctors are in control of their vaginal health. Many women may seek a doctor for issues such as infertility; however, man-made chemicals aren't proving to be useful. Women may have to seek several treatments like hormone therapy. However, natural herbs can balance a woman's hormones naturally, without chemicals or surgery. Unfortunately, there has been an attack on this method of womb healing, especially online via negative or false articles, simply because it actually works!

Although the vagina is self-cleaning, it must be in optimal health in order to do so. If the vagina were in optimum health, women wouldn't experience infertility. Also, there are certain issues that the vagina could not cleanse itself of, such as a cyst or unreleased uterine lining. Unfortunately, our diets also affect hormones more than we know! For example, obesity has also been a cause of infertility as women have been told by their doctors. Still, issues like PCOS can also cause excessive weight gain.

Emotional health and stress can also cause hormonal imbalances. Based on the information provided previously, we know now that hormonal imbalances, in the brain as well, can cause irregular cycles, endometriosis, PCOS, and ultimately infertility. Doctors have started using birth control to assist with PCOS or other vaginal issues caused by hormonal imbalances. Birth control (IUD, Depo Shot, pills) can also affect our bodies negatively. With long-term use, birth control can cause issues with reproducing in the future. Birth control can also have negative effects on hormones as well. Many women may even experience severe mood swings.

How can Yummy Yoni Pearls help me conceive?

Yummy Yoni Pearls contain potent, all-natural herbs that help balance hormones and remove blockage. The blend of herbs supports vaginal health by strengthening the uterus, regulating absent or infrequent cycles. The mix of herbal ingredients is absorbed into the body vaginally to expel contents that may be preventing the vagina from functioning normally. The herbs concentrate on the lower abdomen to help flush and drain the lymphatic system as well.

Yummy Yoni Pearls' blend of herbs can detox your womb and reset your natural balance to improve fertility. The active ingredients include the following:

1. Motherwort – This is a traditional herb used for heart conditions, irregular heartbeat, or heart symptoms due to anxiety and depression. However, motherwort is also utilized for the absence of menstrual periods, flatulence, and hyperthyroidism or overactive thyroid. Motherwort also stimulates uterine tone, blood flow, and reduces menopausal symptoms.

2. Osthol – A type of bicyclic aromatic compound found in many plants. With the research that has been done with osthol, it shows that this substance plays a significant role in liver health, brain function, and dilation of blood vessels.
3. Angelica – A plant. The seed, root, and fruit are used to make medicine. It is used for heartburn, flatulence, loss of appetite, arthritis, circulation problems, nervousness, insomnia. Angelica can also be used to start menstrual periods. Angelica is also useful in increasing urine production as well as to stimulate output and secretion of phlegm, improve sex drive, and kill germs.
4. Borneol – Borneol has a broad range of uses. It occurs naturally in plants such a thyme. Borneol can be used to promote relaxation and reduce exhaustion.

Success stories with Yummy Yoni Pearls

Yummy Yoni Pearls are designed to regulate the menstrual cycle, resulting in shorter, lighter, less painful periods! This cleanse will even cause menstruation in women who have not seen a cycle in years. The blend of herbs also drains cysts and removes excessive or dead vaginal tissue.

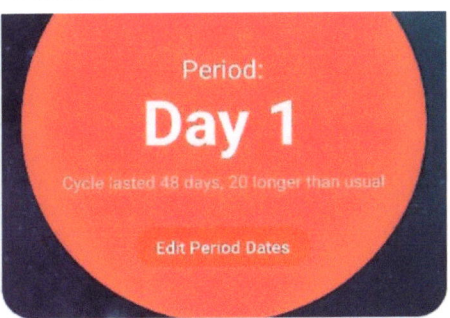

 I think the detox started my cycle

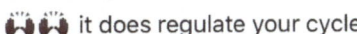 it does regulate your cycle.

 And that's my 2nd detox

Ok cool, are you noticing a difference in your cycles yet?

It's lighter, not heavy at all you're amazing @YUMMYYONIPEARLS

YUMMYYONIPEARLS.NET

Black Seed Oil #Lifeinacan

To maintain or repair your reproductive system, we suggest our 100% natural Black Seed Oil. The Black seed oil is ideal for women who have suffered reproductive damage or scarring. Using just the Black Seed Oil, women have been known to conceive! The Black Seed Oil will also increase sex drive in both sexes. Also, Black Seed Oil can boost sperm count and act as a detox for men as well.

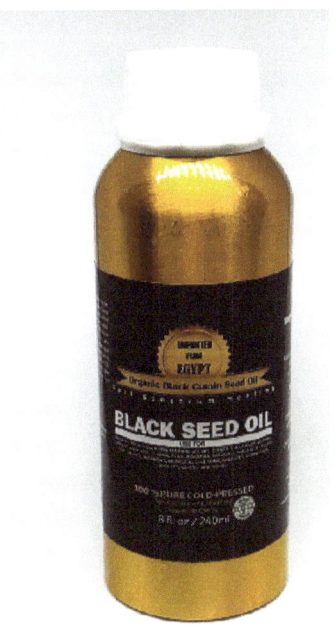

Wanna say thanks to your black seed oil I'm not expecting my first baby 👶 thanks so much I'll keep you posted   @yummyyonipearls

      Not expecting? Or expecting?

Expecting lol sorry typo

Three positive tests super happy thanks so much
      @yummyyonipearls

      Pregnant after only using the oil?

Yes after only taking the oil for month twice a day
      @yummyyonipearls

🤣 💥 👊🏿 OMG! Congrats 😭 so happy for you 🙌🏽 this is why we do this 🥰

Thanks so so much I'll update you as soon as I know how far along I am and even send you pics

YUMMYYONIPEARLS.NET

Tips To Conceive Naturally

1. Cleanse your womb with Yummy Yoni Pearls. To conceive, insert your Yummy Yoni Pearls 10 days before your expected cycle. The goal is to increase fertility before the fertile window. For the best results, cleanse once a month until a cycle is absent. Also, for women with irregular cycles, start cleansing with Yummy Yoni Pearls at any time. More than likely, the Yummy Yoni Pearls will bring on an absent or irregular cycle. If so, simply remove the Yummy Yoni Pearls and wear pads. The vagina will still detox for the remaining 6 days. Downloading a period tracker app makes tracking your cycle and fertile days easy.

2. Take our Black Seed Oil daily to build your immune system. As stated previously, Black Seed Oil has many benefits for both women and men. Actually, the entire family can experience the overall benefits of our Black Seed Oil.

3. The most effective time to have sex is during your fertile window, which can last up to six days every month. These six days are the five days leading up to, and the day of, ovulation. An egg will survive for about a day once released. However, sperm can survive for up to a week inside the womb, so there is a six-day window for sperm to wait for and then meet an egg. You are most likely to conceive if you have sex within a day or so of ovulation. However, it's tricky to pinpoint the exact day or two just before ovulation. Therefore, try to enjoy sex every

two or three days. If you want to be more precise, though, you will need to work out when you will ovulate.

4. Prepare your body for a successful pregnancy. Change your diet, take walks, treat your body as if you're already pregnant. Kick any unhealthy habits like drinking, smoking, or drugs. Get yourself to a healthy weight and limit your caffeine intake to about 16 ounces of coffee a day. For both men and women, food and fertility are linked. Stick to a balanced diet to boost your chances of a healthy baby. Eat several servings of fruit, vegetables, whole grains, and plenty of water. Not getting enough nutrients can affect your periods, making it difficult to predict when you will ovulate. Your partner should also pay attention to his diet since certain vitamins and nutrients—such as zinc and vitamins C and E and folic acid—are important for making healthy sperm. Managing your weight if underweight or obese is vital as well. Plan for a healthy pregnancy.

5. Begin taking folic acid at least one month before you start trying to conceive. This nutrient can dramatically reduce the risk of certain birth defects. Also, taking a prenatal vitamin ensures that you're getting enough folic acid and other essential nutrients to boost your chances of conceiving a healthy baby.

6. Don't wait to have sex until your most fertile time. Your partner should ejaculate at least once in the days just before your most fertile period. Otherwise, there could be a buildup of dead sperm in his semen.

Tips To Conceive Naturally

7. Note that most vaginal lubricants like store-bought products, as well as homemade versions like olive oil, can slow down sperm. If you want to use vaginal lubricants, try a natural product like coconut oil.
8. Reduce stress and negative energy. Relax and follow the tips to conceive naturally.

To learn more about James & James, LLC, products, visit YummyYoniPearls.net. Follow us on Instagram @YummyYoniPearls and like our Yummy Yoni Pearls Facebook fan page.

Yummy Yoni Mommies & Babies!

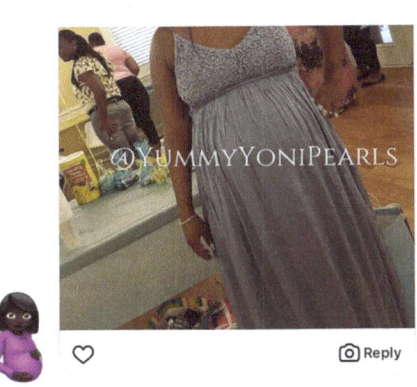

@YummyYoniPearls 🤣 😍 😭

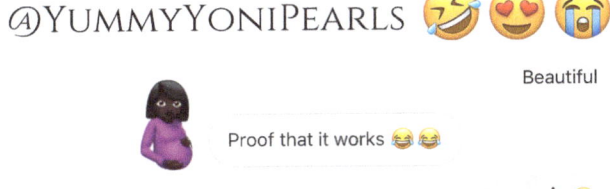

YummyYoniPearls.net

YummyYoniPearls.net | Written by Jared & Mesi James

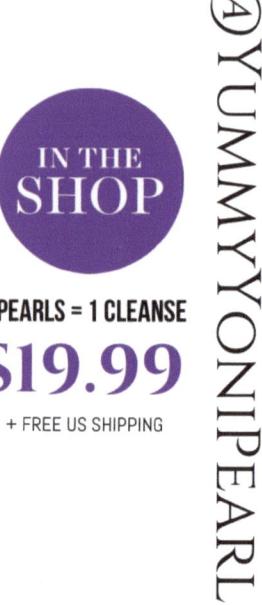

IN THE SHOP

3 PEARLS = 1 CLEANSE

$19.99

+ FREE US SHIPPING

@YUMMYYONIPEARLS

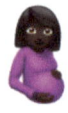 Definitely will ready for that baby

JAN 18, 11:39 AM

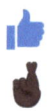

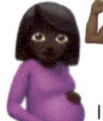 I'm 5 weeks pregnant

MAR 29, 11:08 PM

MAR 30, 1:14 PM

I did the pearls went to the Doc yesterday and confirmed thru blood being drawn and a urine test. I only did one detox only left them in 2 days, the second day wasn't even a full 24 hrs

 Thank you sooooo much

APR 3, 10:40 AM

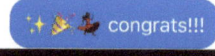

YummyYoniPearls.net

Yummy Yoni Mommies & Babies!

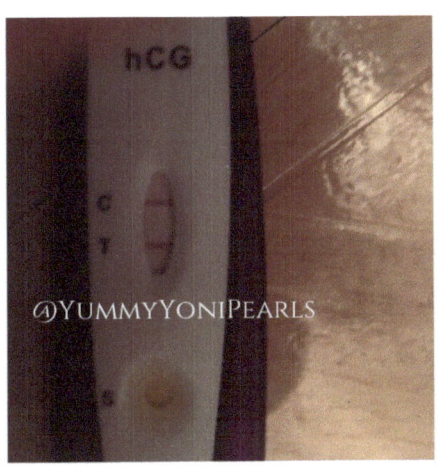

 📷 Reply

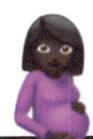 Stop taking my BC of 10 years Feb 25th cleansed that same week and just found out today im 6 weeks pregnant!!! Wasn't expecting it to happen SO DAMN QUICK still shocked @YummyYoniPearls

YummyYoniPearls.NET

YummyYoniPearls.net | Written by Jared & Mesi James

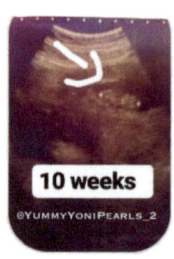

YUMMYYONIPEARLS.NET

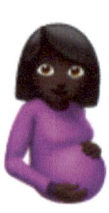

I've had issues in the past with pregnancies not getting past 7 weeks. I used yummy yoni pearls once. And now my doctor tells me it's a slim chance of miscarriage this time. Thanks Queens ... For having a product that really works. @YUMMYYONIPEARLS_2

Omg! My eyes are watering 😭😍 Congrats Goddess! Thank you for trusting me!

Yummy Yoni Mommies & Babies!

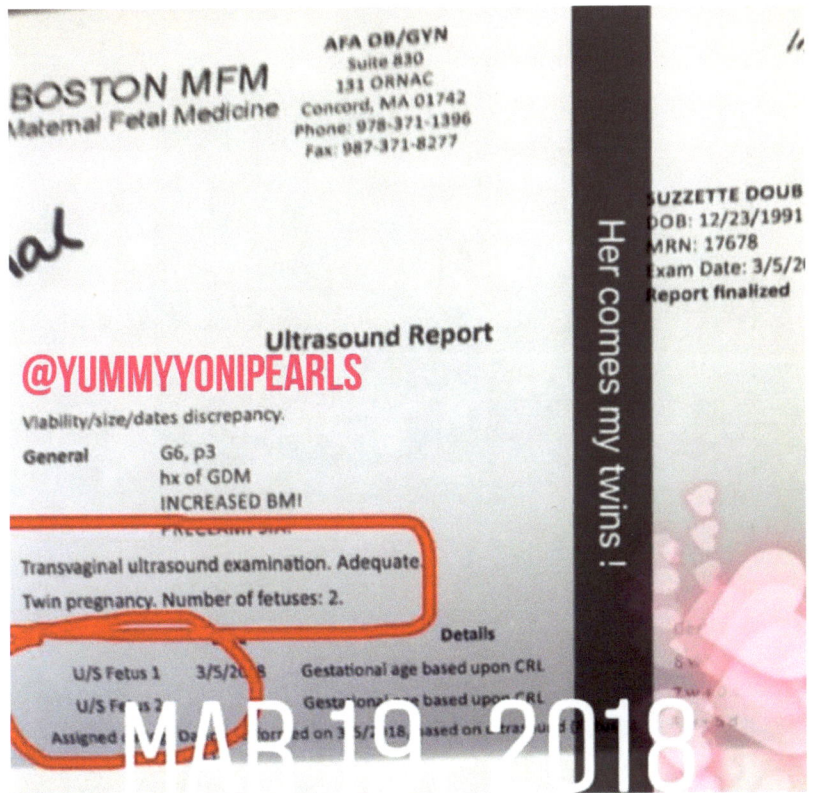

YummyYoniPearls.net | Written by Jared & Mesi James

I'm almost a week late
@YummyYoniPearls

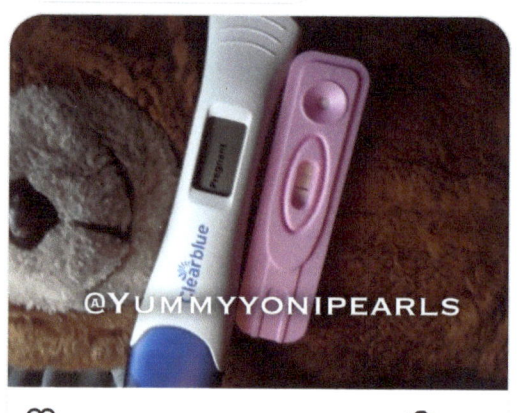

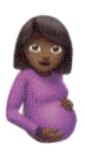

No and congrats 🎉 how long have you been trying to get pregnant?

@YummyYoniPearls
I have not got pregnant in 5 years

YummyYoniPearls.net

Yummy Yoni Mommies & Babies!

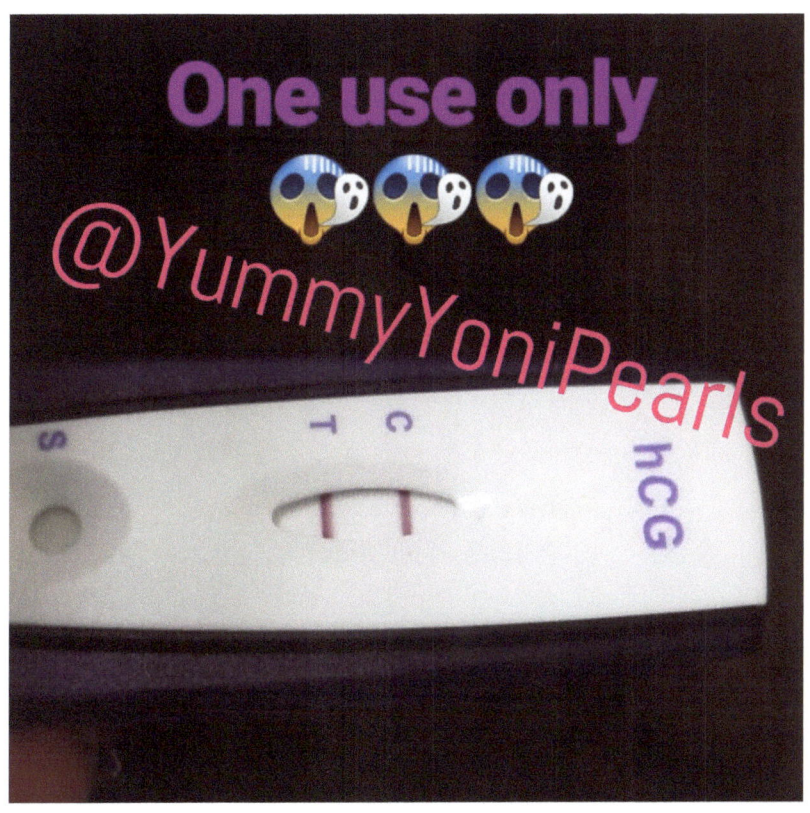

YummyYoniPearls.net | Written by Jared & Mesi James

I have been trying for 2 years in finally finally i just tried your product n it worked!! Very blessed
@YummyYoniPearls

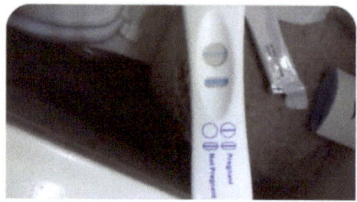

♡   📷 Reply

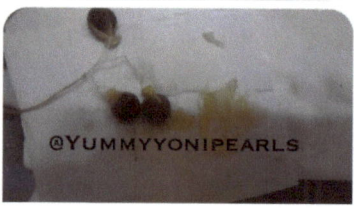

♡   📷 Reply

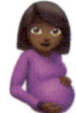 I detoxed n november had a perfect period december n here it is January 18 n i am pregnant im still in disbelief
@YummyYoniPearls

YummyYoniPearls.net

Yummy Yoni Mommies & Babies!

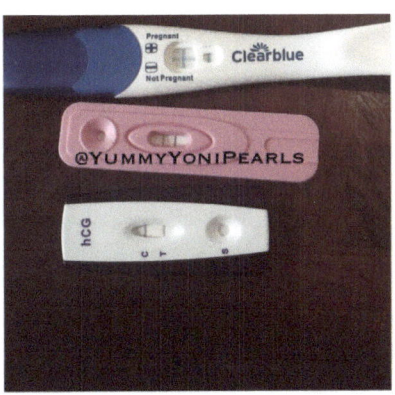

 I can't thank you enough 😭😭

Omg 😭 how many cleanses?

 I did two cleanses. I have PCOS and we've been trying for 4 years. Spent last year on fertility meds that didn't work at all.

YUMMYYONIPEARLS.NET

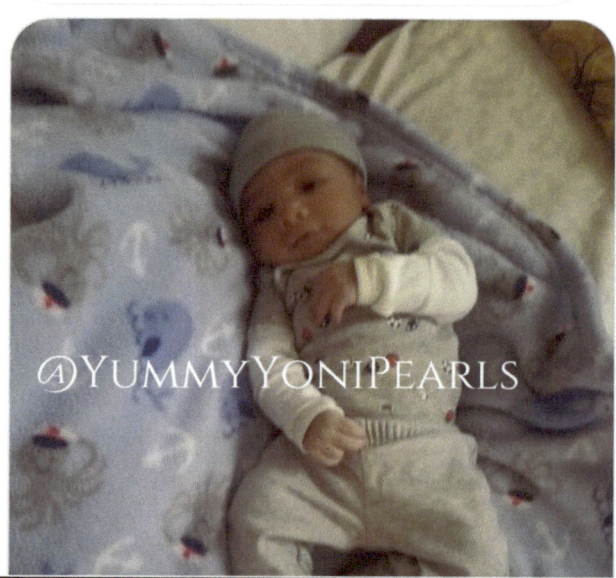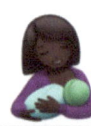

Yummy Yoni Mommies & Babies!

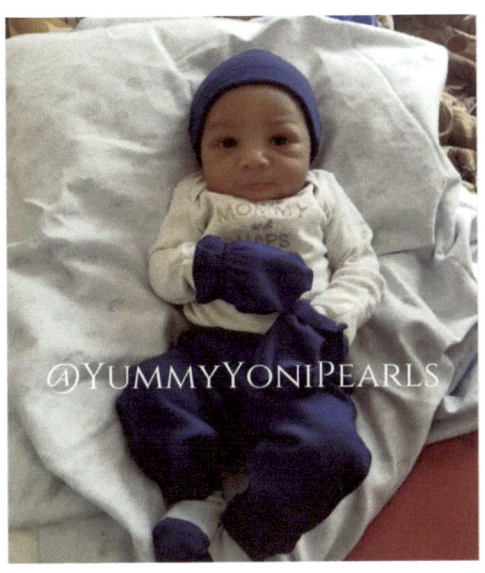

A week old sunday

YUMMYYONIPEARLS.NET

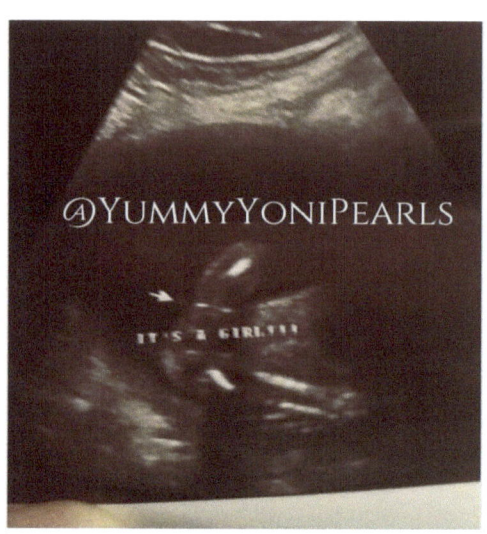

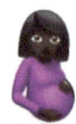 These pearls change lifes completely!! #Blessed

YUMMYYONIPEARLS.NET

Yummy Yoni Mommies & Babies!

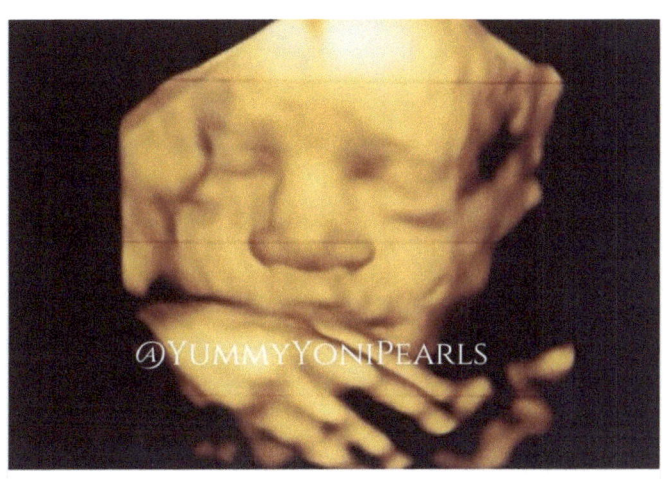

 @YummyYoniPearls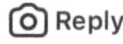

 6 more weeks to go and he will be here 🙌🏻🙌🏻🙌🏻🙌🏻🙌🏻❤️💋💋

YummyYoniPearls.net

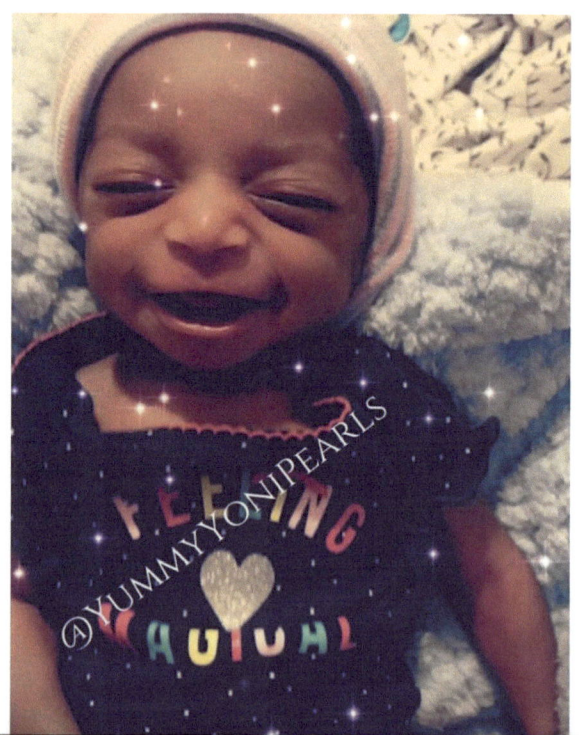

Yummy Yoni Mommies & Babies!

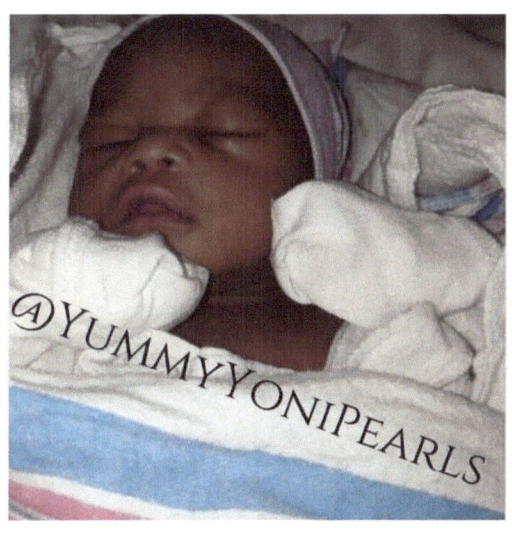

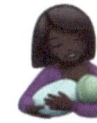
Here's your yummiyonipearls baby
@YummyYoniPearls

YummyYoniPearls.net

All of the success stories, photos, and testimonies in this guide are 100% authentic. See more by following on Instagram @YummyYoniPearls. Yummy Yoni Pearls are just one of the many herbal products sold and manufactured by James & James, LLC.

James & James, LLC, was established by the Founder, Jared James, in 2014. Yummy Yoni Pearls is just one of Jared's many online brands which have grown into stores! After his wife and the C.E.O. of James & James, LLC, Mesi James, experienced her first detox, Jared encouraged Mesi to share her story. With more research and the help of distant relatives, the James' were ready to create their own brand of yoni pearls. In early 2017, Jared & Mesi launched Yummy Yoni Pearls.

The James' have other branches of James & James, LLC, including The Photo Shop, Atlanta. Their products include Charcoal Tooth Powder, Black Seed Oil, Yummy Yoni Eggs, and other services/products. The James' also give love and business advice in their books, **Young, Black, & Married: How to Snuggle thru the Struggle** and **Young, Black, & Married: Teamwork makes the Dream Work.** To learn more about all the products and services offered by James & James, LLC, visit JamesandJamesLLC.com. To learn more about the James' book and DVD series, visit YoungBlackandMarried.net.

Yummy Yoni Mommies & Babies!

Follow all the James & James, LLC, brands on Instagram @charcoaltoothpowder, @yummyyonipearls, @wearethejames, @VagicSticks, @PrettyKittyBoutique, @YummyYoniEggs, and @_thephotoshop_. The goal of James & James, LLC, is to rebuild Black Wall Street one brick at a time, starting with the family! Visit our other websites to shop all James & James, LLC, products:

ThePhotoShop.net

PrettyKittyBoutique.net

www.ingramcontent.com/pod-product-compliance
Lightning Source LLC
Chambersburg PA
CBHW040245220526
45473CB00001B/379